IMPROVE YOUR HEALTH WITH

BREATHWORK

The practical breathwork exercise that stops anxiety & stress, boost energy, & promotes optimal wellness & lots more + frequent questions and answers

BY,

DOCTOR WEALTH SNOW

Copyright@2021

TABLE OF CONTENT

CHAPTER ONE

DESCRIBING BREATHWORK

In case you're keen on taking a stab at breathing activities to lessen pressure or uneasiness, or improve your lung work, nitty gritty activities are recorded underneath for you to harness.

You may locate that specific activities appeal to you immediately. Start with the training that is agreeable to you.

The most effective method to add breathing activities to your daily living are listed below. Breathing activities don't need to remove a great deal of time from your day. It's truly pretty much putting aside some an ideal opportunity to focus on your relaxing. Follow the below listed steps.

- Start with only 5 minutes per day, and increment your time as the activity gets simpler and more agreeable.
- On the off chance that 5 minutes feels excessively long, start with only 2 minutes.
- Practice on various occasions a day. Timetable set occasions or practice cognizant breathing as the need arises.

Advantages of Breathing Exercises

- It brings stress and anxiety to a reduced level
- Breathing Exercises increment our oxygen admission and quiet our psyche. They are demonstrated to be exceptionally powerful in decreasing pressure and tension.
- It enhances the quality of sleep
- **Breathing activities loosen up our body and quiet down our brain.** They assist us with disposing of pressure and nervousness. Breathing activities subsequently help us in getting a decent night rest.
- **It improves Cognitive Functions**

- Performing breathing activities as often as possible improves fixation and core interest

Additionally, our memory and dynamic capacities are improved upon.

- **Improvement in Cardiovascular Health:**

Performing Breathing activities regularly helps in keeping up our pulse levels and assists patients with hypertension. The occurrence of Stroke and heart illnesses is decreased.

We can now say that breathing activities is amazingly important in the strengthening of our cardiovascular function.

- **It improves Lungs function:**

Breathing activities help in better functioning of our lungs. They have end up being monstrously helpful for patients with constant lung infections like Asthma, Emphysema, Bronchitis, COPD and so on

- **It Detoxify our body:**

Engaging breathing activities causes our body to dispose harmful gases and carbon dioxide. This process detoxifies our body.

- **Supports Digestive System:**

Performing breathing activities consistently guarantees smooth working our stomach related framework and assists with disposing of gastrointestinal issues like tooting, blockage, swelling, acid reflux and so forth

They likewise give alleviation from side effects of GERD (Gastroesophageal Reflux Disease).

- **Give a Glow to our Skin:**

Breathing activities like pranayama increment the inventory of oxygen, which expands the blood thrush and improves the presence of skin. It additionally detoxifies blood which brings about more youthful and gleaming skin.

- **Fight Sinusitis:**

Breathing Exercises help in the therapy of persistent sinusitis.

- Help in Weight Loss:

Breathing Exercises enact our abs.

- Improve Immunity:

Breathing Exercises improve the protection system of our body, in this way boosting insusceptibility.

- **Anti-maturing:**

Breathing activities help in hindering the maturing interaction.

They help to keep up body weight, forestall wrinkles and keep skin sparkling, decrease pressure, reinforce muscular strength, right awful stance and so on.

CHAPTER TWO

LIST OF BREATHING TECHNIQUES

Below is some list of breathing techniques;

1) TIGHTENED LIP RELAXING
2) DIAPHRAGMATIC RELAXING
3) BREATH CENTER PROCEDURE
4) LION'S BREATH
5) SUBSTITUTE NOSTRIL RELAXING
6) EQUIVALENT RELAXING
7) RESOUNDING OR INTELLIGIBLE RELAXING
8) SITALI BREATH
9) PROFOUND RELAXING
10) MURMURING HONEY BEE BREATH (bhramari)

1. TIGHTENED LIP RELAXING

This basic breathing procedure makes you hinder your speed of breathing by having you apply conscious exertion in every breath.

You can rehearse pressed together lip breathing whenever. It could be particularly helpful during exercises, for example, bowing, lifting, or step climbing.

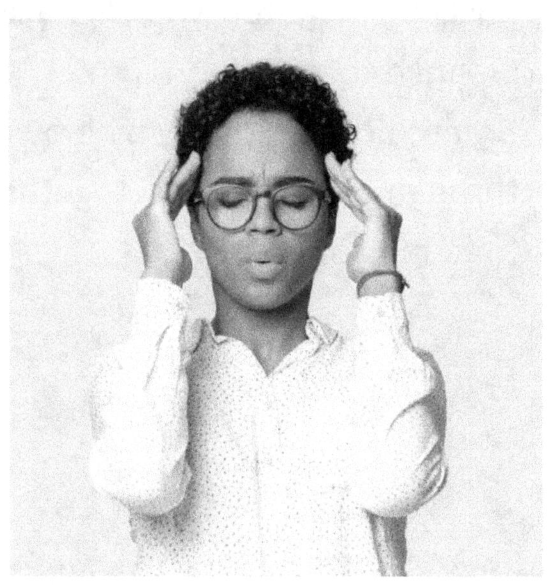

Work on utilizing this breath 4 to 5 times each day when you start to effectively become familiar with the breathing example.

To do it:

- ✓ Loosen up your neck and shoulders.
- ✓ Keeping your mouth shut, breathe in gradually through your nose for 2 checks.
- ✓ Pucker or tighten your lips like you planned to whistle.
- ✓ Breathe out gradually by blowing air through your pressed together lips for a tally of 4.

2. DIAPHRAGMATIC RELAXING

Tummy breathing can help you utilize your stomach appropriately. Do gut breathing activities when you're feeling loose and rested.

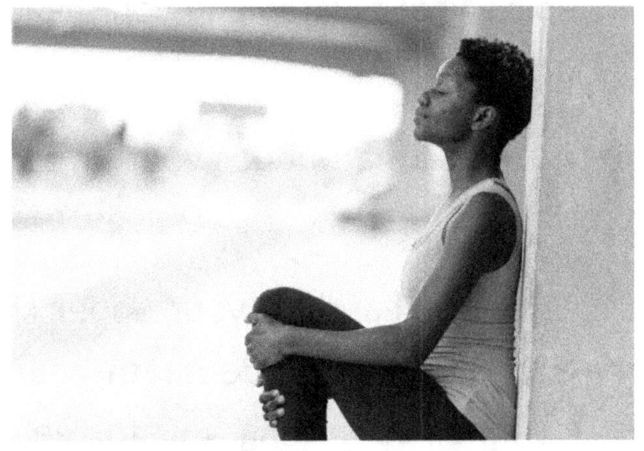

Practice diaphragmatic relaxing for 5 to 10 minutes 3 to 4 times each day.

At the point when you start you may feel tired, however after some time the procedure ought to get simpler and should feel more regular.

To do it:

✓ Lie on your back with your knees somewhat twisted and your head on a cushion.

You may put a pad under your knees for help.

✓ Spot one hand on your upper chest and one hand underneath your rib confine, permitting you to feel the development of your stomach.

✓ Gradually breathe in through your nose, feeling your stomach squeezing into your hand.

✓ Keep your other hand as still as could be expected.

✓ Breathe out utilizing pressed together lips as you fix your stomach muscles, keeping your advantage totally still.

✓ You can put a book on your mid-region to make the activity more troublesome.

When you figure out how to do midsection breathing resting you can expand the trouble by attempting it while sitting in a seat. You would then be able to rehearse the strategy while playing out your every day exercises.

3. BREATH CENTER PROCEDURE

This profound breathing procedure utilizes symbolism or center words and expressions.

You can pick a center word that makes you grin, feel loose, or that is just unbiased to consider. Models incorporate harmony, let go, or unwind, yet it tends to be any word that suits you to zero in on and rehash through your training.

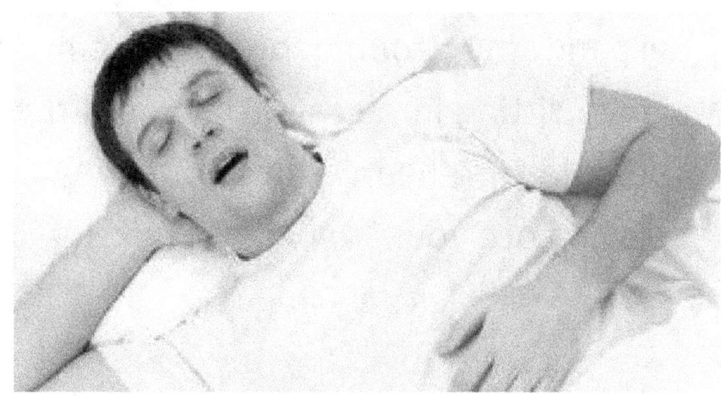

As you develop your breath center practice you can begin with a 10-minute meeting. Progressively increment the span until your meetings are in any event 20 minutes.

To do it:

✓ Sit or rests in an agreeable spot.

✓ Carry your attention to your breaths without attempting to change how you're relaxing.

✓ Switch back and forth among ordinary and full breaths a couple of times. Notice any contrasts between typical breathing and profound relaxing. Notice how your midsection extends with profound inward breaths.

Note how shallow breathing feels contrasted with profound relaxing.

- ✓ Practice your profound relaxing for a couple of moments.
- ✓ Spot one hand beneath your paunch button, keeping your midsection loose, and notice how it ascends with each breathe in and falls with each breathe out.
- ✓ Let out a noisy murmur with each breathe out.

Start the act of breath center by joining this profound breathing with symbolism and a center word or expression that will uphold unwinding.

You can envision that the air you breathe in brings floods of harmony and quiet all through your body.

Envision that the air you breathe out washes away strain and nervousness

4. LION'S BREATH

Lion's breath is an empowering yoga breathing practice that is said to diminish pressure in your chest and face.

It's additionally referred to in yoga as Lion's Pose or simhasana in Sanskrit.

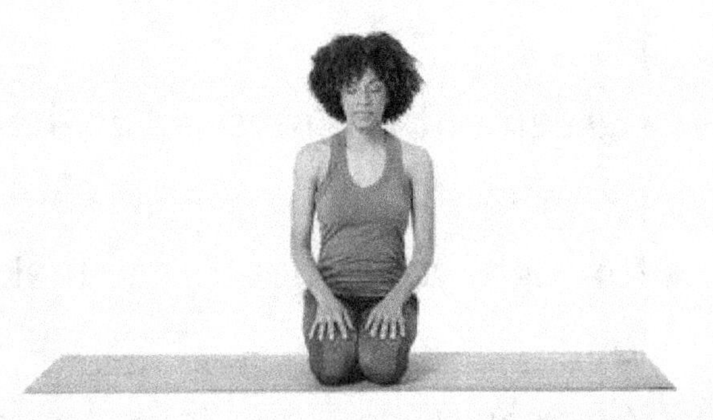

To do this:

✓ Come into an agreeable situated position. You can sit out of sorts or fold your legs.

- ✓ Make sure your palm is press against the knees with the finger widely spread apart.
- ✓ Breathe in profoundly through your nose and make sure the eyes are widely open.
- ✓ Simultaneously, open your mouth wide and stick out your tongue, bringing the tip down toward your jaw.
- ✓ Agreement the muscles at the front of your throat as you breathe out through your mouth by making a long "ha" sound.
- ✓ You can turn your look to take a gander at the space between your eyebrows or the tip of your nose.

Do this breath 2 to multiple times.

5. SUBSTITUTE NOSTRIL RELAXING

Substitute nostril breathing, known as nadi shodhana pranayama in Sanskrit, is a breathing practice for unwinding.

Substitute nostril breathing has been appeared to upgrade cardiovascular capacity and to bring down pulse.

Nadi shodhana is best rehearsed on an unfilled stomach. Evade the training in case you're feeling debilitated or clogged. Keep your breath smooth and even all through the training.

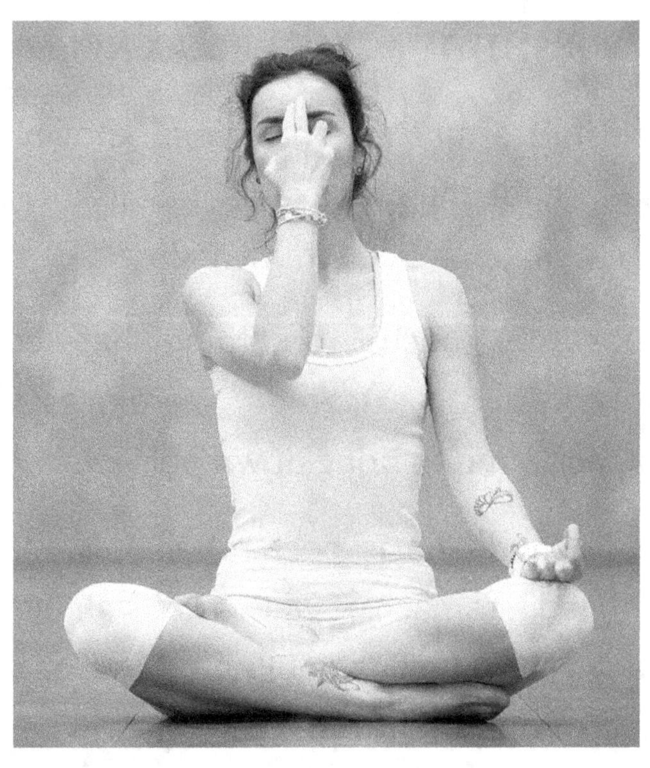

To do this:

- ✓ Pick an agreeable situated position.
- ✓ Lift up your correct hand toward your nose, squeezing your first and center fingers down toward your palm and leaving your different fingers broadened.

✓ After a breath out, utilize your correct thumb to delicately close your correct nostril.

Breathe in through your left nostril and afterward close your left nostril with your correct pinky and ring fingers.

✓ Delivery your thumb and breathe out through your correct nostril. Breathe in through your correct nostril and afterward close this nostril.

✓ Delivery your fingers to open your left nostril and breathe out through this side.

This is one cycle.

Proceed with this breathing example for as long as 5 minutes.

Finish your meeting with a breath out on the left side.

6. EQUIVALENT RELAXING

The term "Equivalent breathing" may also be refers to as sama vritti. This breathing procedure centers around making your breathes in and breathes out a similar length. Making your breath smooth and consistent can help achieve equilibrium and serenity.

Engage the breath length that is simple so as to stay clear from trouble. You likewise need it to be too quick, so that you're ready to keep up it all through the training.

When you become accustomed to rise to breathing while situated you can do it during your yoga practice or other every day exercises.

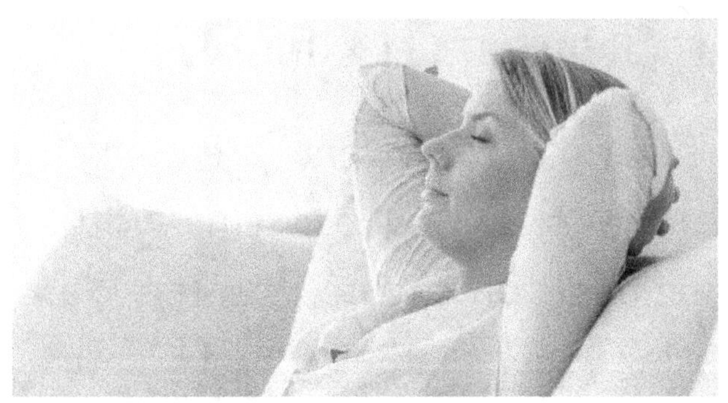

To do it:

- ✓ Pick an agreeable situated position.
- ✓ Take in and out through your nose.
- ✓ Tally during each breathe in and breathe out to ensure they are even in term. On the other hand, pick a word or short expressions to continue during each breathe in and breathe out.
- ✓ You can add a slight delay or breathe maintenance after each breathe in and breathe out in the event that you feel great. (Ordinary

breathing includes a characteristic respite).

Continue this process up to 5 times.

7. RESOUNDING OR INTELLIGIBLE RELAXING

Resounding breathing, otherwise called intelligent breathing, is the point at which you inhale at a pace of 5 full breaths each moment. You can accomplish this rate by breathing in and breathing out for a check of 5.

Breathing in light of present conditions expands your pulse inconstancy (HRV), decreases pressure, and diminish indications of discouragement when joined with Iyengar yoga.

To do this:

- ✓ Breathe in for 5 consecutive times.
- ✓ Breathe out for 5 consecutive times.

Proceeds with this breathing example for at any rate a couple of moments.

8. SITALI BREATH

This yoga breathing practice causes you bring down your internal heat level and loosen up your psyche.

Marginally broaden your breath long yet don't compel it. Since you breathe in through your mouth during Sitali breath, you might need to pick a spot to rehearse that is liberated from any allergens that influence you and air contamination.

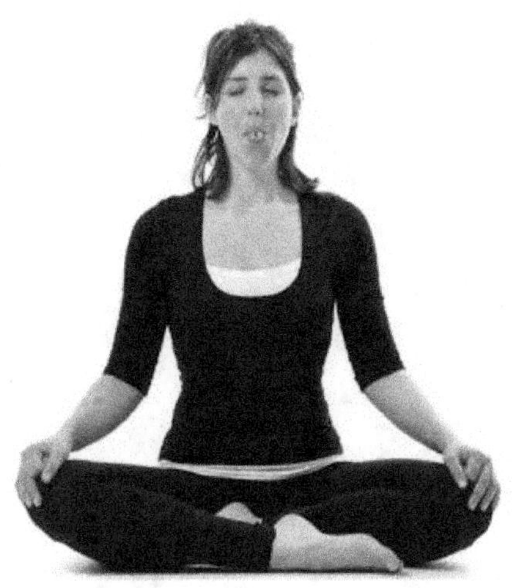

To do this:

- ✓ Pick an agreeable situated position.
- ✓ Stick out your tongue and twist your tongue to unite the external edges. In the event that your tongue doesn't do this, you can press together your lips.
- ✓ Breathe in through your mouth.
- ✓ Breathe out through your nose. Continue this process up to 5 times.

9. PROFOUND RELAXING

Profound breathing assists with mitigating windedness by keeping air from getting caught in your lungs and assisting you with taking in more natural air. It might assist you with feeling more loose and focused.

To do this:

- ✓ While standing or sitting, step your elbows back marginally to permit your chest to grow.
- ✓ Take a profound inward breath through your nose.
- ✓ Hold your breath for a tally of 5.
- ✓ Gradually discharge your breath by breathing out through your nose.

10. MURMURING HONEY BEE BREATH (bhramari)

The novel impression of this yoga breathing practice assists with making moment quiet and is particularly mitigating around your temple. A few people use murmuring honey bee breath to diminish disappointment, tension, and outrage. Obviously, you'll need to rehearse it in where you are allowed to make a murmuring sound.

To do this:

- ✓ Pick an agreeable situated position. You can now close your eyes with your face loosen up.
- ✓ Spot your first fingers on the tragus ligament that incompletely covers your ear waterway.

- ✓ Breathe in, and as you breathe out delicately press your fingers into the ligament.
- ✓ Keeping your mouth shut, make a boisterous murmuring sound.
- ✓ Proceed however long is agreeable.

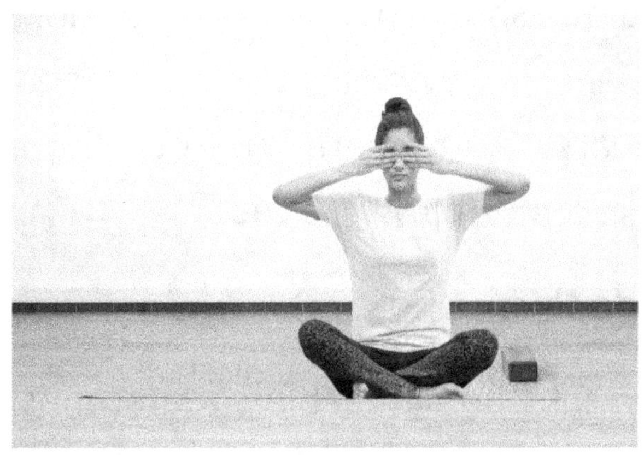

CHAPTER THREE

a) Why should I learn breathing techniques?

It is good you learn breathing techniques because you might be breathing wrongly thereby not oxygenating the body for better impact.

b) Why is a personal coach good in learning breathwork?

This is because it is difficult to attend to group at a time and figure out their challenges rather a one on one coaching is better. Some people are slow learners which makes them far from the teaching of the day.

c) Does a breathe coaches has former training and full certification?

Yes, from a teacher training colleges.

d)   Who should not practice breathwork?

- Children who are not guided by a specialist.
- Person who suffers cardiac arrhythmia, heart block, and persons taking antipsychotic medication.
- Tell the doctor about your present health condition before engaging breathwork.

e)   How long will it take to positively feel the impact of breathwork?

It's base on individual differences because some takes a week to see the impact while others a month. How well you engaged the exercise determines how fast you get the result.

CONCLUSION

You can attempt the vast majority of these breath practices immediately. Set aside the effort to explore different avenues regarding various kinds of breathing procedures. Devote a specific measure of time in any event a couple of times each week. You can do these activities for the duration of the day.

Check in with your PCP on the off chance that you have any clinical concerns or take any drugs. In the event that you need to become familiar with breathing practices you can counsel a respiratory advisor or a yoga educator who has some expertise in breathing practices. Stop the training in the event that you experience any sensations of uneasiness or unsettling.

You will enjoy all the benefits of breath work if you follow the entire guide written in this book.

THE END